I0479961

TRAINING YOUR DOG FOR A HAPPY LIFE

My Journey with Max

Williams Bryant

Table of Content

Introduction

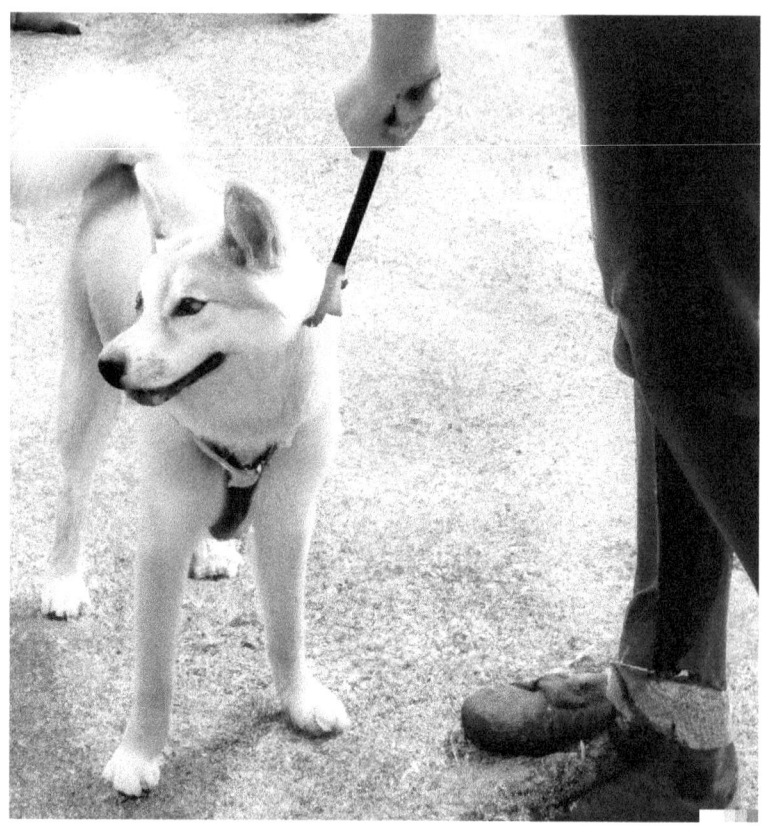

I had always been a cat person. Growing up, my family had a few felines, and I loved their independent personalities and sassy attitudes. I never really saw the appeal of dogs. They seemed loud, needy, and a bit too eager for attention.

That was until I met Max. Max was a golden retriever, and he belonged to a friend of a friend. I wasn't particularly excited when my friend invited me over to hang out with her and her dog, but I figured it would be a good opportunity to socialize.

When I arrived, Max was lying on the living room rug, his tail wagging lazily. My friend introduced us, and Max immediately got up and approached me. He sniffed my hand and then nudged his head under my palm; as if to say hello. I was surprised by how gentle and friendly he was. He didn't jump on me or bark incessantly as I had expected. Instead, he seemed content to sit by my side and listen as I talked to my friend.

Over the next few hours, Max and I became fast friends. I found myself laughing at his goofy expressions and marveling at his intelligence. He seemed to understand me in a way that no other animal had before.

As the evening wore on, I realized that I had been wrong about dogs. They weren't just loud and needy; they were loyal, affectionate, and intuitive. Max had won me over, and I knew that I would never be a cat person again.

Since that day, Max and I have been inseparable. We go on long walks, cuddle on the couch, and play fetch in the park. He's my constant companion, and I couldn't imagine my life without him. Max has taught me that dogs are more than just pets; they're family. They have a special ability to understand and comfort us, even when we don't know we need it. And for that, I am forever grateful.

The Nature of Dogs

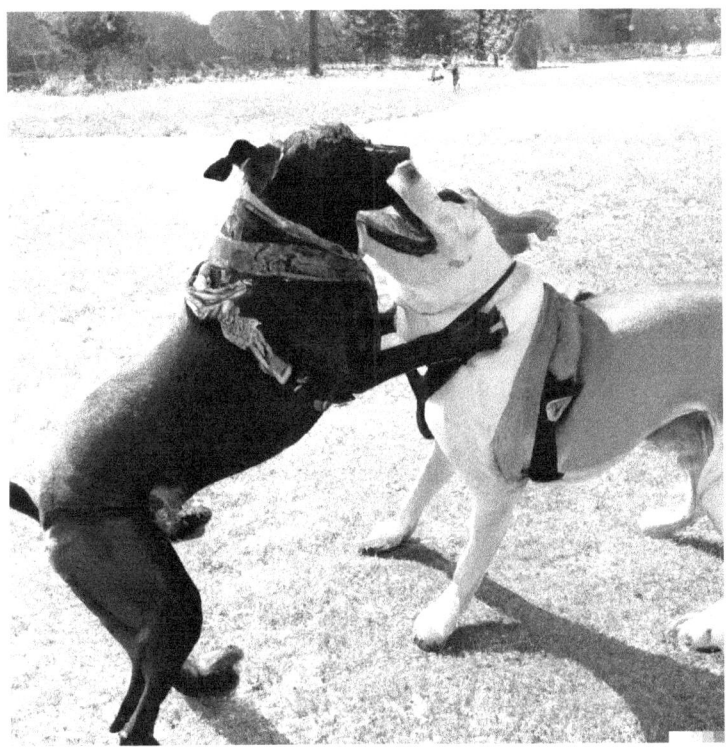

I woke up to the sound of my alarm clock blaring, signaling the start of another day. As I dragged myself out of bed, I was greeted by the enthusiastic wagging of my dog's tail. I couldn't help but smile as I scratched him behind the ears and he leaned into me, his warm body pressing against my leg.

As I got ready for the day ahead, my dog followed me from room to room, never leaving my side. It was like he knew I needed his companionship to face whatever challenges the day may bring. And he was right. As I stepped out into the world, I was immediately hit by a wave of stress and anxiety. But with my furry friend by my side, I felt a sense of calm wash over me. His presence was a constant reminder that no matter what happened, I wasn't alone.

Throughout the day, my dog continued to be my faithful companion. He greeted me with wagging tail and slobbery kisses when I returned home from work, and he snuggled up to me on the couch as I decompressed from the day's events.

But it wasn't just his constant presence that made my dog the best companion. It was also his unwavering loyalty and unconditional love. No matter how many mistakes I made or how bad of a day I was having, my dog never judged me. He was always there with a wagging tail and a happy bark, reminding me that I was loved and accepted just the way I am.

As the years went by, my dog continued to be my constant companion, always by my side through the good times and the bad. And as I looked into his trusting eyes, I knew that I had found the best companion a person could ask for. So if you ever find yourself feeling alone or lost, just remember that there's a furry friend out there waiting to be your loyal companion. Because when it comes to finding a true companion, there's nothing quite like the love and loyalty of a dog.

Dogs are one of the most beloved animals on the planet, known for their loyalty, affectionate nature, and playful personalities. They are commonly referred to as "man's best friend" and are often considered as part of the family in many households. But what makes dogs so special, and what is the nature of these furry creatures?

To understand the nature of dogs, it is essential to examine their evolutionary history. The domestication of dogs occurred over 15,000 years ago, when wolves began to interact with early human settlements. Over time, these wolves evolved into the dogs that we know and love today, developing unique traits and characteristics that set them apart from their wild counterparts.

One of the most notable traits of dogs is their sociability. Dogs are packed animals, and their social nature makes them highly responsive to human interaction. They have evolved to read human cues, such as body language and vocal cues, and respond to them accordingly. This makes dogs excellent companions and loyal protectors, as they form strong bonds with their owners and become an integral part of their families.

Another key aspect of a dog's nature is its intelligence. Dogs are highly trainable and can learn a variety of tasks and commands, from basic obedience to complex tricks and tasks. They are also adept at problem-solving and can use their senses to navigate their environment and find solutions to challenges they encounter.

Despite their domestication, dogs still retain some of their wild instincts. They have a natural prey drive, and many breeds are excellent hunters. They also have a strong sense of smell, which they use to track scents and identify objects and people. This has led to the development of breeds specifically trained for tasks such as hunting, search and rescue, and law enforcement.

Dogs are known for their emotional intelligence. They are capable of a range of emotions, from joy and excitement to fear and sadness. Dogs have been shown to respond to human emotions, displaying empathy and offering comfort when their owners are upset or distressed. This emotional connection between dogs and humans is a significant part of what makes them such popular and beloved pets.

Dogs are particularly attuned to the emotions and body language of their human companions, and they can often pick up on subtle cues that other animals or even humans may miss. For example, a dog may be able to sense when their owner is feeling anxious or stressed, and they may respond by offering physical affection or calming behavior. Similarly, dogs can recognize when their owners are feeling happy or playful, and they may respond with their own displays of excitement and joy.

One reason for dogs' high emotional intelligence may be their long history of domestication and close relationship with humans. Over thousands of years of domestication, dogs have evolved to be highly attuned to human behavior and emotions. In many ways, they have become experts at reading our body language and facial expressions, and they are able to respond to our emotional cues in ways that other animals cannot.

In addition to their emotional intelligence, dogs are also valued for their loyalty, companionship, and ability to provide a sense of security and safety to their human companions. They are often considered members of the family, and many people feel a deep emotional connection with their dogs that is similar to the connection they have with other human beings. Dogs have been domesticated for thousands of years and have evolved alongside humans, developing a unique bond with us that is difficult to replicate with any other animal.

One of the reasons dogs are so valued for their loyalty is that they are pack animals by nature. In the wild, dogs form tight-knit social groups and rely on each other for survival. This social structure has carried over into domesticated dogs, who often see their human families as their pack. They are instinctively wired to be loyal and protective of their pack members, which is why they make such great companions and protectors.

Dogs also provide a sense of security and safety to their human companions. They have keen senses and are often used as guard dogs to protect homes and businesses. Even small dogs can be trained to alert their owners to potential threats, such as strangers approaching the home or unusual noises. This ability to provide a sense of security and protection is especially important for people who live alone or who are vulnerable, such as the elderly or those with disabilities.

Finally, the emotional connection that people feel with their dogs is difficult to quantify but is no less real. Dogs have been shown to have a calming effect on their owners and can even help alleviate symptoms of depression and anxiety. They are always there to provide comfort and companionship, no matter what mood their owner is in. This emotional connection is often what makes dogs such an important part of their owner's lives and why they are considered members of the family.

Types of Dogs

Dogs are one of the most diverse and beloved animals in the world. There are hundreds of different breeds of dogs, each with their own unique characteristics and traits. Here we'll explore some of the most popular types of dogs and what makes them special.

- Labrador Retriever - This is one of the most popular breeds in the world and is known for their friendly and outgoing nature. Labradors are often used as service dogs, therapy dogs, and guide dogs for the blind because of their intelligence, obedience, and loyalty. They are also great family pets because they are gentle and patient with children.
- German Shepherd - German Shepherds are highly intelligent and trainable dogs that are often used as police and military dogs. They are known for their courage, loyalty, and protective nature, which makes them excellent guard dogs. German Shepherds are also loyal family pets that love to be active and enjoy spending time with their owners.
- Golden Retriever - Golden Retrievers are friendly, outgoing dogs that are known for their loyalty and love of people. They are often used as therapy dogs because of their gentle and calming nature. Golden Retrievers also make great family pets because they are patient with children and love to play.
- Bulldog - Bulldogs are known for their unique appearance and laid-back nature. They are often referred to as the "clowns" of the dog world because of their goofy personalities. Bulldogs make great

family pets because they are affectionate and love to cuddle.

- Chihuahua - Chihuahuas are small dogs with big personalities. They are often referred to as "purse dogs" because they are small enough to be carried around in a purse. Chihuahuas are loyal and protective of their owners, which makes them great watch dogs. They are also good apartment dogs because they don't require a lot of space or exercise.
- Poodle - Poodles are highly intelligent and trainable dogs that come in three different sizes: standard, miniature, and toy. They are often used in dog shows because of their unique appearance and fancy haircuts. Poodles make great family pets because they are affectionate and love to be around people.
- Boxer - Boxers are energetic and playful dogs that are known for their love of people. They are often used as therapy dogs because of their gentle nature. Boxers make great family pets because they are patient with children and love to play.
- Beagle - Beagles are friendly and curious dogs that are known for their love of sniffing. They are often used as hunting dogs because of their keen sense of smell. Beagles make great family pets because they are affectionate and love to play.
- Rottweiler - Rottweilers are loyal and protective dogs that are often used as guard dogs. They are known for their strength and courage, which makes them excellent protectors. Rottweilers also make great family pets because they are affectionate and loyal to their owners.

- Siberian Husky - Siberian Huskies are energetic and playful dogs that are known for their love of running. They are often used as sled dogs because of their strength and endurance. Siberian Huskies make great family pets because they are affectionate and love to play.

The Labrador Retriever

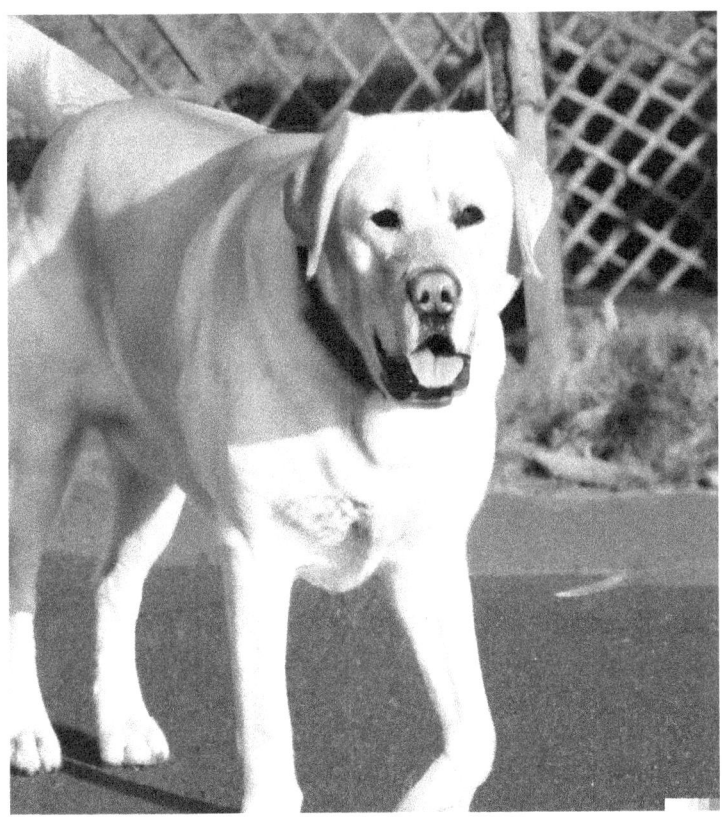

The Labrador Retriever is one of the most beloved dog breeds in the world. These dogs are known for their friendly and outgoing nature, intelligence, and loyalty. In this article, we will explore some of the unique characteristics of the Labrador Retriever and why they are such popular pets.

The Labrador Retriever originated in Newfoundland, Canada, in the 1700s. These dogs were originally bred to help fishermen retrieve fish that had fallen off hooks or escaped from nets. Over time, the Labrador Retriever became popular with hunters because of their ability to retrieve game from both water and land. Today, the Labrador Retriever is one of the most popular breeds in the world and is often used as service dogs, therapy dogs, and guide dogs for the blind.

The Labrador Retriever is a medium to large-sized dog that can weigh between 55 and 80 pounds. They have a short, dense coat that comes in three colors: yellow, black, and chocolate. Their ears hang down and their tails are thick and powerful. The Labrador Retriever has a muscular build and a friendly expression.

The Labrador Retriever is known for its friendly and outgoing nature. They are affectionate and love to be around people, which makes them great family pets. They are also intelligent and trainable, which makes them popular with service dog organizations. The Labrador Retriever is patient with children and other animals, which makes them a great choice for families with kids or other pets.

One of the Labrador Retriever's greatest strengths is their ability to retrieve. They have a soft mouth, which means they can retrieve game without damaging it. This makes them popular with hunters and also makes them great at playing fetch. The Labrador Retriever is also a great swimmer and loves to be in the water. They have webbed feet that help them paddle, which makes them great at retrieving items from the water.

Another strength of the Labrador Retriever is their intelligence. They are highly trainable and are often used as service dogs, therapy dogs, and guide dogs for the blind. They are also great at obedience training and can learn a wide range of commands.

The Labrador Retriever is generally a healthy breed, but like all dogs, they can be prone to certain health problems. Some of the health issues that can affect Labrador Retrievers include hip and elbow dysplasia, eye problems, and obesity. It's important to keep your Labrador Retriever at a healthy weight and to provide them with regular exercise to help prevent health problems.

The Labrador Retriever is a unique and beloved breed of dog. They are friendly, outgoing, intelligent, and loyal, which makes them great family pets and working dogs. Whether you are looking for a companion or a service dog, the Labrador Retriever is an excellent choice.

However, as with any dog, it's important to do your research and make sure the Labrador Retriever is the right breed for your lifestyle and needs.

The German Shepherd

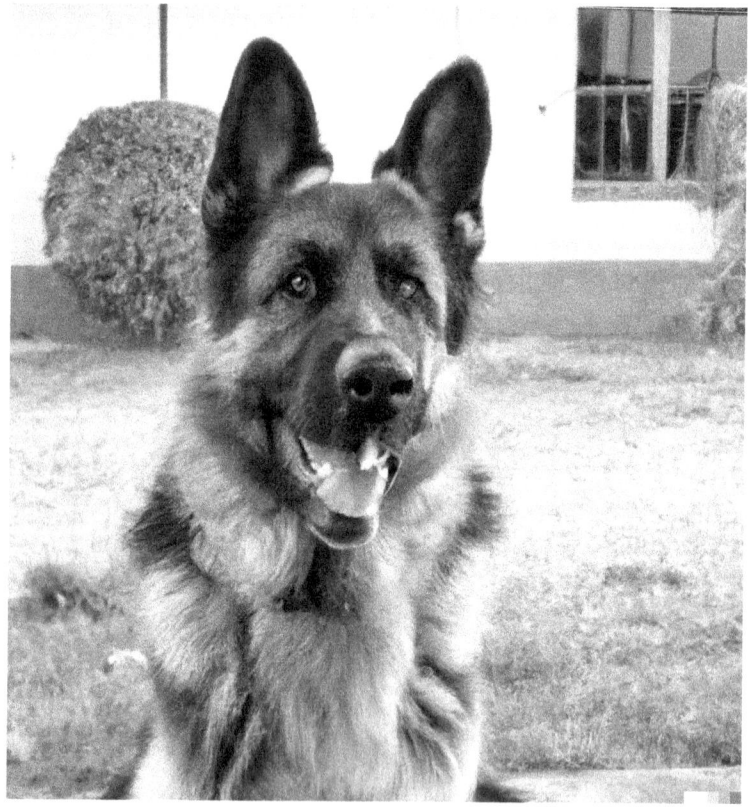

The German Shepherd is a breed of dog that is known for its intelligence, loyalty, and strength. These dogs are often used as working dogs in law enforcement, military, and search and rescue organizations, as well as family pets.

The German Shepherd was first developed in Germany in the late 19th century. The breed was created by Captain Max von Stephanitz, who wanted to create a dog that was versatile, trainable, and loyal. The German Shepherd was originally used as a herding dog, but over time, they became popular with law enforcement agencies and the military because of their intelligence, strength, and loyalty.

The German Shepherd is a medium to large-sized dog that can weigh between 50 and 90 pounds. They have a double coat that is thick and dense, and they come in a variety of colors, including black and tan, black and red, and solid black. Their ears are erect and their tails are long and bushy. The German Shepherd has a muscular build and a confident and alert expression.

The German Shepherd is known for its intelligence, loyalty, and protectiveness. They are highly trainable and are often used as police dogs, search and rescue dogs, and guide dogs for the blind. They are also great family pets and are known for their loyalty and protectiveness towards their owners. The German Shepherd is a confident and courageous dog, but they can also be reserved with strangers.

One of the German Shepherd's greatest strengths is their intelligence. They are highly trainable and are often used as working dogs because of their ability to learn and carry out complex tasks. They are also great at obedience training and can learn a wide range of commands.

Another strength of the German Shepherd is their strength and athleticism. They are powerful dogs that have a lot of energy, which makes them great at activities like running, hiking, and playing fetch. They are also great at protecting their owners and their homes, which makes them popular with families.

The German Shepherd is generally a healthy breed, but like all dogs, they can be prone to certain health problems. Some of the health issues that can affect German Shepherds include hip and elbow dysplasia, bloat, and skin problems. It's important to keep your German Shepherd at a healthy weight and to provide them with regular exercise to help prevent health problems.

The German Shepherd is a unique and beloved breed of dog. They are intelligent, loyal, and protective, which makes them great working dogs and family pets. Whether you are looking for a companion or a working dog, the German Shepherd is an excellent choice. However, as with any dog, it's important to do your research and make sure the German Shepherd is the right breed for your lifestyle and needs.

The Golden Retriever

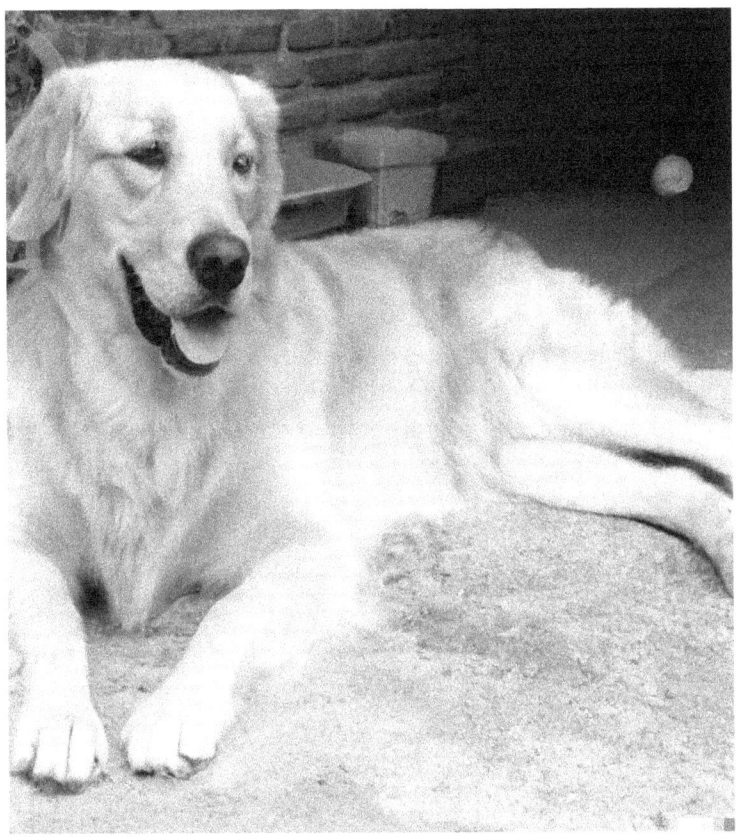

The Golden Retriever is a beloved breed of dog known for its friendly personality, intelligence, and loyalty. They are often considered the quintessential family dog and are popular pets all around the world.

The Golden Retriever was originally bred in Scotland in the mid-19th century. The breed was created by a

Scottish aristocrat named Sir Dudley Marjoribanks, who wanted to develop a dog that was able to retrieve game from land and water. The breed was initially called the Golden Flat-Coat, but eventually, the name was changed to the Golden Retriever. Today, the Golden Retriever is a popular breed in the United States, where they are often used as hunting dogs, family pets, and service dogs.

The Golden Retriever is a medium to large-sized dog that can weigh between 55 and 75 pounds. They have a thick, water-repellent coat that is typically golden in color, and their ears are medium-sized and pendant-shaped. The Golden Retriever has a muscular build and a friendly, intelligent expression.

The Golden Retriever is known for its friendly and outgoing personality. They are highly social dogs and are great with children and other pets. They are also highly intelligent and easy to train, which makes them popular with families and as service dogs. The Golden Retriever is also known for their loyalty, and they are often protective of their owners.

One of the Golden Retriever's greatest strengths is their intelligence. They are highly trainable and are often used as service dogs because of their ability to learn and carry out complex tasks. They are also great at obedience training and can learn a wide range of commands.

Another strength of the Golden Retriever is their athleticism. They are active dogs that require a lot of exercise, which makes them great at activities like running, swimming, and playing fetch. They are also great at retrieving and can be trained to retrieve items from land and water.

The Golden Retriever is generally a healthy breed, but like all dogs, they can be prone to certain health problems. Some of the health issues that can affect Golden Retrievers include hip and elbow dysplasia, cancer, and skin problems. It's important to keep your Golden Retriever at a healthy weight and to provide them with regular exercise to help prevent health problems.

The Golden Retriever is a unique and beloved breed of dog. They are friendly, intelligent, and loyal, which makes them great family pets and service dogs. Whether you are looking for a companion or a working dog, the Golden Retriever is an excellent choice. However, as with any dog, it's important to do your research and make sure the Golden Retriever is the right breed for your lifestyle and needs.

Bulldog

The Bulldog, also known as the English Bulldog, is a unique and recognizable breed of dog that is known for its stout and muscular appearance. Despite its intimidating appearance, the Bulldog is actually a gentle and affectionate breed that is great with children and families.

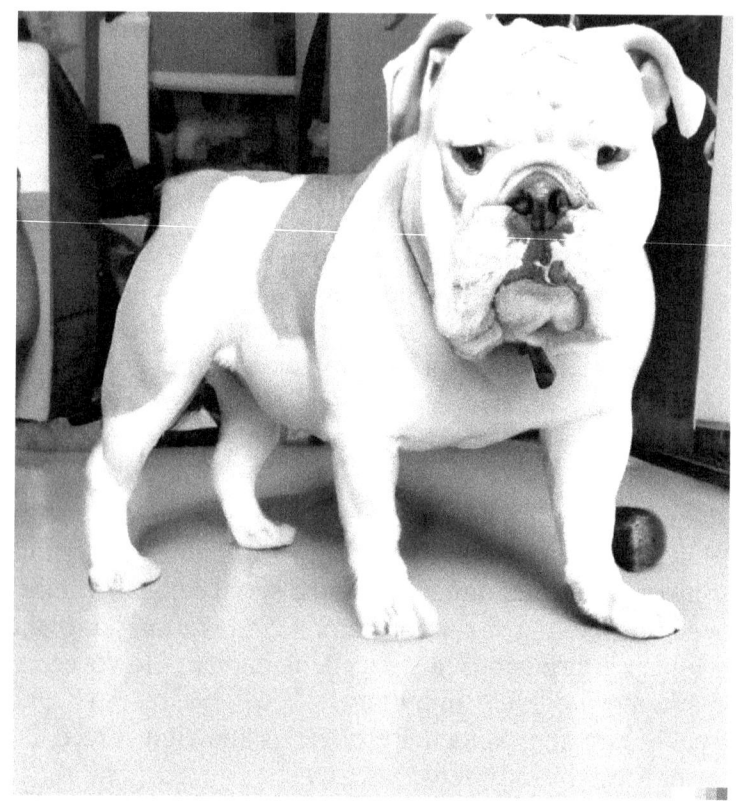

The Bulldog was originally bred in England for bull-baiting, a cruel sport that was outlawed in the 19th century. After bull-baiting was banned, the Bulldog was bred to be a companion dog and its aggressive tendencies were bred out of it. Today, the Bulldog is a popular breed around the world and is known for its friendly and loyal personality.

The Bulldog is a medium-sized dog that typically weighs between 40 and 50 pounds. They have a stocky, muscular build and a large, wrinkled head with a short, wide muzzle. Their coat is short and comes in a variety of colors, including white, brindle, and fawn.

The Bulldog is a gentle and affectionate breed that is great with children and families. They are loyal and protective of their owners, but they are not aggressive. Bulldogs are known for their stubborn streak, but they are also intelligent and trainable. They are not particularly active dogs and prefer to spend their time lounging with their owners.

One of the Bulldog's greatest strengths is their loyalty. They are devoted to their owners and will do anything to protect them. They are also known for their courage and will stand up to larger dogs or even intruders if they perceive a threat to their family.

Another strength of the Bulldog is their adaptability. They can thrive in both urban and rural environments and are comfortable in apartments or large homes. They do not require a lot of exercise and are content with a short walk or play session.

The Bulldog is a generally healthy breed, but like all dogs, they can be prone to certain health problems. Some of the health issues that can affect Bulldogs include hip dysplasia, breathing problems, and skin allergies. It's important to keep your Bulldog at a healthy weight and to provide them with regular exercise to help prevent health problems.

The Bulldog is a unique and lovable breed of dog. They are great with families and children and are known for their loyalty and protective instincts. Whether you are looking for a companion or a guard dog, the Bulldog is an excellent choice. However, as with any dog, it's important to do your research and make sure the Bulldog is the right breed for your lifestyle and needs.

Chihuahuas

Chihuahuas are a unique breed of dog that is known for their small size, distinctive appearance, and spunky personality. Despite their diminutive stature, Chihuahuas are packed with energy and have a remarkable strength that belies their size.

The Chihuahua breed originated in the state of Chihuahua in Mexico, which is where they got their name. The breed is believed to have descended from the Techichi dog, a small companion dog that was kept by the Toltec people in ancient Mexico. Chihuahuas were first brought to the United States in the late 19th century, where they quickly gained popularity as a fashionable lapdog.

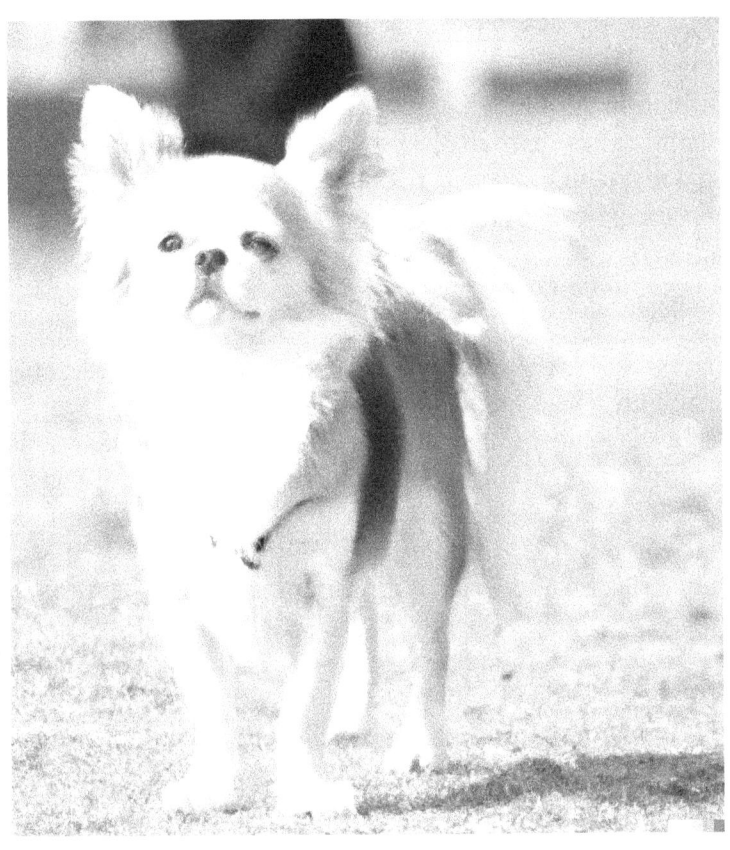

Chihuahuas are the smallest breed of dog, with an average height of 6-10 inches and weight ranging from 2-6 pounds. They have a distinctive "apple" shaped head and large, round eyes that give them a perpetually surprised expression. Chihuahuas come in a variety of colors and patterns, including black, white, fawn, chocolate, and brindle.

Despite their small size, Chihuahuas are known for their big personalities. They are energetic, playful, and affectionate dogs that are fiercely loyal to their owners. Chihuahuas are also known for being stubborn and independent, which can make them difficult to train at times. They have a tendency to be protective of their owners, which can lead to them being territorial or aggressive towards strangers.

Despite their tiny size, Chihuahuas have a remarkable strength and athleticism that can surprise many people. They are incredibly agile and quick, with a remarkable ability to jump and climb. Chihuahuas have been known to jump up to five times their own height, and can run at speeds of up to 18 miles per hour. Their small size also makes them ideal for agility training, as they can easily navigate obstacles and tight spaces.

Like all breeds of dog, Chihuahuas are susceptible to certain health issues. Some of the most common health concerns for Chihuahuas include dental problems, hypoglycemia, patellar luxation, and heart disease. It's important for Chihuahua owners to keep up with regular vet checkups and maintain a healthy diet and exercise routine for their dogs.

Chihuahuas are a unique and beloved breed of dog that has captured the hearts of many people around the world. Their small size, big personality, and remarkable athleticism make them an ideal companion for those looking for a loyal and energetic pet. Despite their occasional stubbornness and territorial tendencies,

Chihuahuas are incredibly loving and affectionate dogs that can bring joy to any household.

Poodles

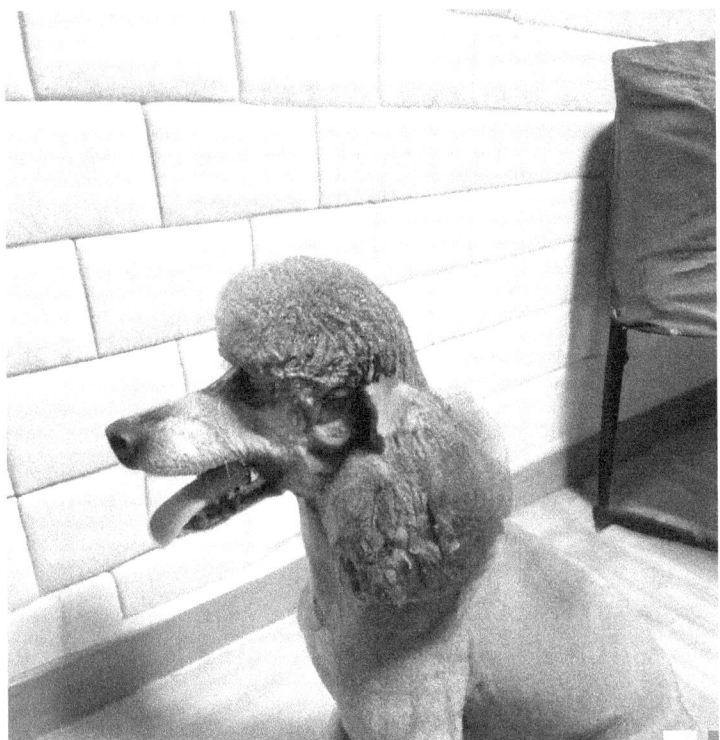

Poodles are a popular breed of dog that are known for their distinctive curly coat, intelligence, and versatility. They are one of the oldest dog breeds, with a history that dates back to the 15th century.

Poodles are believed to have originated in Germany, where they were bred as water retrievers for hunting. They were later popularized in France, where they became a fashionable companion dog for the aristocracy. Poodles come in three sizes - Standard, Miniature, and Toy - and can be found in a variety of colors, including black, white, brown, and apricot.

Poodles are known for their distinctive curly coat, which is hypoallergenic and does not shed. This makes them an ideal breed for people with allergies. Their coat is also incredibly dense and requires regular grooming to prevent matting. Poodles are a muscular and athletic breed, with an elegant appearance that belies their working dog origins.

Poodles are highly intelligent dogs that are known for their trainability and adaptability. They are affectionate and loving dogs that thrive on human companionship. Poodles are also very social dogs that get along well with children and other pets. They have a playful and energetic personality, but are also capable of being calm and relaxed when they need to be.

Poodles are a highly athletic breed of dog that excel in a variety of sports and activities. They were originally bred as water retrievers, which means they have a natural instinct for swimming. Poodles are also known for their agility and are often trained for sports such as agility, obedience, and flyball. Their intelligence and trainability also make them an ideal breed for service work, such as search and rescue or therapy dog work.

Like all breeds of dog, Poodles are susceptible to certain health issues. Some of the most common health concerns for Poodles include hip dysplasia, eye problems, and skin allergies. It's important for Poodle owners to keep up with regular vet checkups and maintain a healthy diet and exercise routine for their dogs.

Poodles are a versatile and beloved breed of dog that have captured the hearts of many people around the world. Their distinctive curly coat, intelligence, and athleticism make them an ideal companion for those looking for a trainable and adaptable pet. Despite their occasional health concerns, Poodles are generally a healthy breed that can bring joy to any household.

Boxers

Boxers are a highly popular and beloved breed of dog that have captured the hearts of many dog lovers worldwide. These dogs are known for their unique appearance, strong personality, and loyal temperament. Here, we'll take a closer look at what makes boxers so special and why they are such a popular breed.

First, let's examine the physical attributes of boxers. These dogs are medium-sized and muscular, with a square, blocky head and a powerful jaw. They have a short, smooth coat that comes in a variety of colors, including brindle, fawn, and white. Boxers are also known for their distinctive droopy jowls and expressive eyes, which give them a highly expressive and charming appearance.

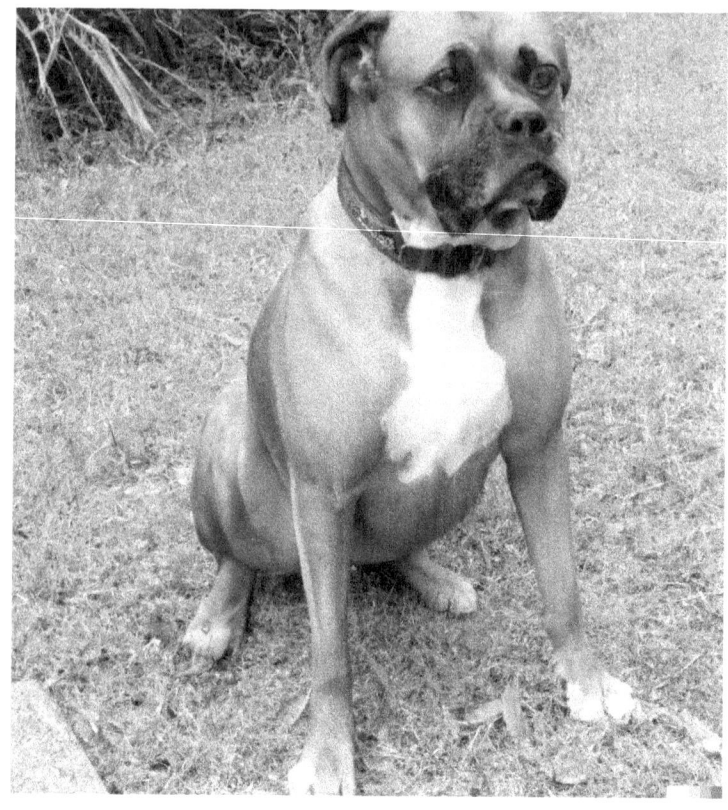

Boxers are also highly active and energetic dogs that require regular exercise and playtime. They are known for their strong, athletic build and agility, which makes them excellent companions for outdoor activities like hiking and running. Boxers are also highly trainable and intelligent, which makes them excellent candidates for obedience and agility training.

But what truly sets boxers apart from other breeds is their loyal and affectionate temperament. Boxers are highly social and love to be around people, which makes them excellent family pets. They are also highly protective of their owners and will go to great lengths to keep them safe. Boxers are known for their love of children and are often described as gentle giants, despite their strong appearance.

One of the unique characteristics of boxers is their playful and sometimes goofy nature. These dogs are known for their love of play and will often engage in silly antics to entertain their owners. Boxers are also highly empathetic and intuitive dogs that can sense their owner's emotions and provide comfort and support when needed.

In terms of health, boxers are generally a robust and healthy breed. However, like all breeds, they are prone to certain health conditions, including hip dysplasia, heart disease, and cancer. Boxers also have a shorter lifespan than some other breeds, with an average lifespan of 8-10 years.

Boxers are a unique and special breed of dog that offer their owners a combination of physical strength, intelligence, loyalty, and affection. They are highly social dogs that thrive in the company of people and are known for their playful and sometimes goofy nature. If you're looking for a loyal and loving companion that can keep up with your active lifestyle, then a boxer may be the perfect breed for you.

Beagles

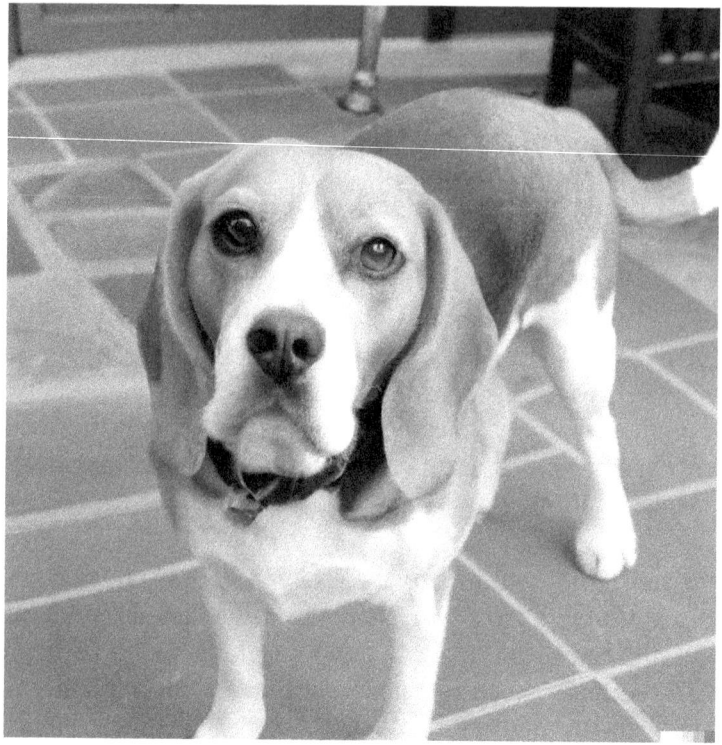

Beagles are a beloved and highly popular breed of dog that are known for their sweet and friendly nature, distinctive looks, and remarkable sense of smell. Here, we'll take a closer look at what makes beagles so special and why they are such a popular breed.

First, let's examine the physical attributes of beagles. These dogs are small to medium-sized with a compact and muscular body. They have a short, smooth coat that comes in a variety of colors, including black, white, tan, and lemon. Beagles are also known for their long, droopy ears and soulful eyes, which give them a charming and endearing appearance.

Beagles are also highly active and energetic dogs that require regular exercise and playtime. They are known for their exceptional sense of smell and were originally bred as hunting dogs to track and chase small game. This means that beagles have a lot of energy and need plenty of exercise to stay healthy and happy. Beagles are also highly trainable and intelligent, which makes them excellent candidates for obedience and agility training.

But what truly sets beagles apart from other breeds is their sweet and friendly temperament. Beagles are highly social dogs that love to be around people and other animals. They are known for their gentle and affectionate nature, which makes them excellent family pets. Beagles are also highly tolerant and patient with children, which makes them a popular choice for families with young kids.

One of the unique characteristics of beagles is their vocal nature. These dogs are known for their distinctive howl, which they use to communicate with their owners and other dogs. Beagles are also highly curious and inquisitive dogs that love to explore their surroundings. This can sometimes get them into trouble, as they are known to follow their nose and wander off if they catch an interesting scent.

In terms of health, beagles are generally a robust and healthy breed. However, like all breeds, they are prone to certain health conditions, including hip dysplasia, ear infections, and obesity. Beagles also have a longer lifespan than some other breeds, with an average lifespan of 12-15 years.

Beagles are a special and unique breed of dog that offer their owners a combination of loyalty, affection, intelligence, and a remarkable sense of smell. They are highly social dogs that thrive in the company of people and other animals and are known for their sweet and friendly nature. If you're looking for a loving and playful companion that can keep up with your active lifestyle, then a beagle may be the perfect breed for you.

Rottweilers
Rottweilers are a breed of large, muscular dogs that have gained a reputation for their strength, intelligence, and loyalty. Originally bred in Germany as a herding dog, the Rottweiler has since become a popular breed for families, law enforcement, and military work.

One of the unique features of the Rottweiler is their physical appearance. They are a medium to large breed with a robust, muscular build that gives them an imposing presence. They typically stand between 22-27 inches tall and weigh between 77-135 pounds. Their coat is short, dense, and black with rust-colored markings on their face, chest, and legs.

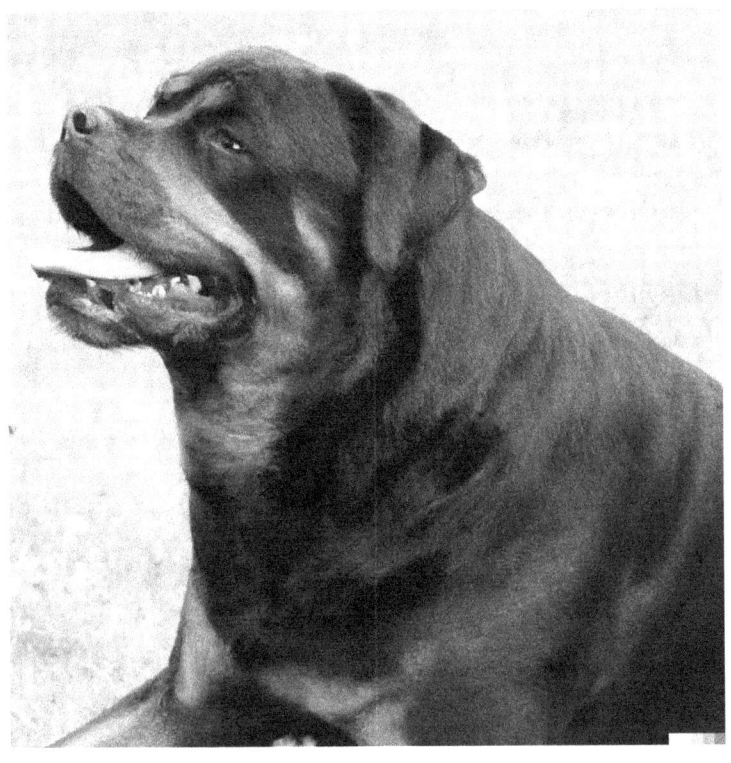

Beyond their physical appearance, Rottweilers are also known for their intelligence and trainability. They are a highly trainable breed that responds well to positive reinforcement and consistent training. They are quick learners and have been used in a variety of roles, including as police dogs, therapy dogs, and service dogs.

Another unique aspect of Rottweilers is their loyalty and protective nature. They have a strong desire to protect their family and can be wary of strangers. With proper socialization and training, however, Rottweilers can be friendly and sociable dogs.

In terms of health, Rottweilers are generally a healthy breed but can be prone to certain health issues. These include hip dysplasia, elbow dysplasia, and bloat. Responsible breeding and regular veterinary care can help minimize the risk of these health concerns.

While Rottweilers have a reputation for being aggressive, this is not necessarily true. Like any breed, Rottweilers can become aggressive if they are not properly trained and socialized. With proper training and socialization, however, Rottweilers can be friendly, well-behaved dogs.

Rottweilers are a unique and powerful breed that can make excellent family pets, as well as working dogs in various fields. With their intelligence, loyalty, and trainability, Rottweilers can excel in a variety of roles and make wonderful companions for those who are willing to put in the time and effort to train and socialize them properly.

Siberian Huskies

Siberian Huskies are an ancient breed of dog that originated in Siberia, Russia. They were bred by the Chukchi people for their strength, endurance, and ability to withstand the harsh arctic climate. Today, they are popular pets and working dogs around the world. Here are some of the unique qualities and strengths that make Siberian Huskies such beloved companions.

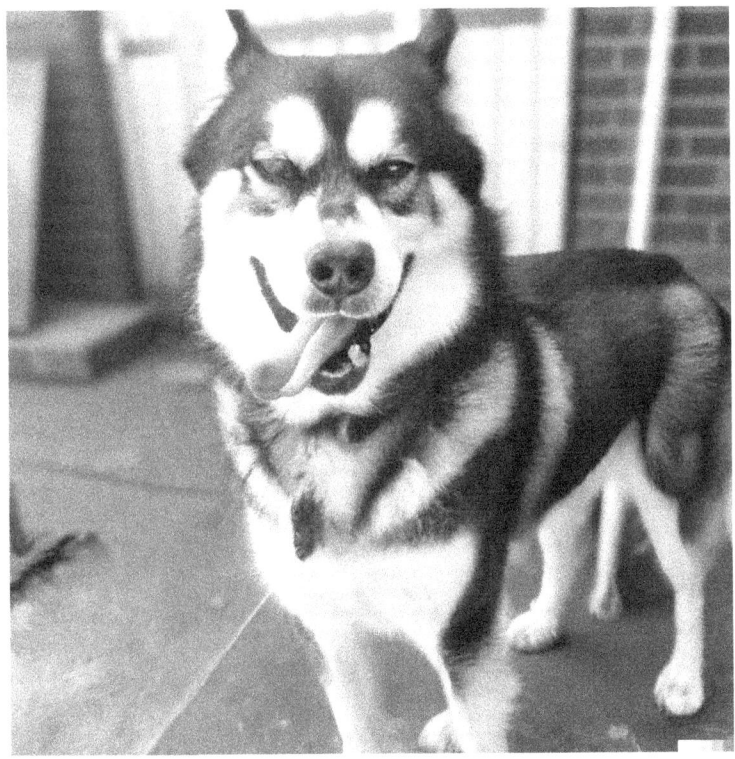

Siberian Huskies are medium-sized dogs that typically weigh between 35 and 60 pounds. They have a thick, double coat that helps protect them from the cold, and they come in a wide variety of colors, including black, white, gray, red, and sable. Their eyes are usually blue or brown, although some dogs have one of each color.

Siberian Huskies are incredibly strong and have a lot of endurance. They were originally bred to pull sleds across vast distances, and they are still used for this purpose today in some parts of the world. Huskies have a unique gait that allows them to move quickly and efficiently, even in deep snow or on rough terrain. They can travel up to 100 miles a day, and they can do it for several days in a row without getting tired.

Siberian Huskies are known for their friendly and outgoing personalities. They are intelligent dogs that are easy to train, and they are great with children and other pets. However, they do have a strong prey drive, so they may not be the best choice for families with small animals. Huskies also have a lot of energy and require plenty of exercise and mental stimulation to be happy and healthy.

Siberian Huskies are generally healthy dogs, but they are prone to a few specific health issues. One of the most common problems is hip dysplasia, which is a condition where the hip joint doesn't develop properly and can cause pain and arthritis. Huskies are also susceptible to eye problems, such as cataracts and progressive retinal atrophy. It's important to have your Husky regularly checked by a veterinarian to catch any health issues early.

Siberian Huskies are a unique and beloved breed of dog that make great pets for the right families. They are strong, intelligent, and friendly dogs that require plenty of exercise and mental stimulation to be happy and healthy. If you're considering adding a Husky to your family, be sure to do your research and find a reputable breeder or rescue organization. With the right care and training, your Husky can be a loyal and loving companion for many years to come.

Training Your Dog

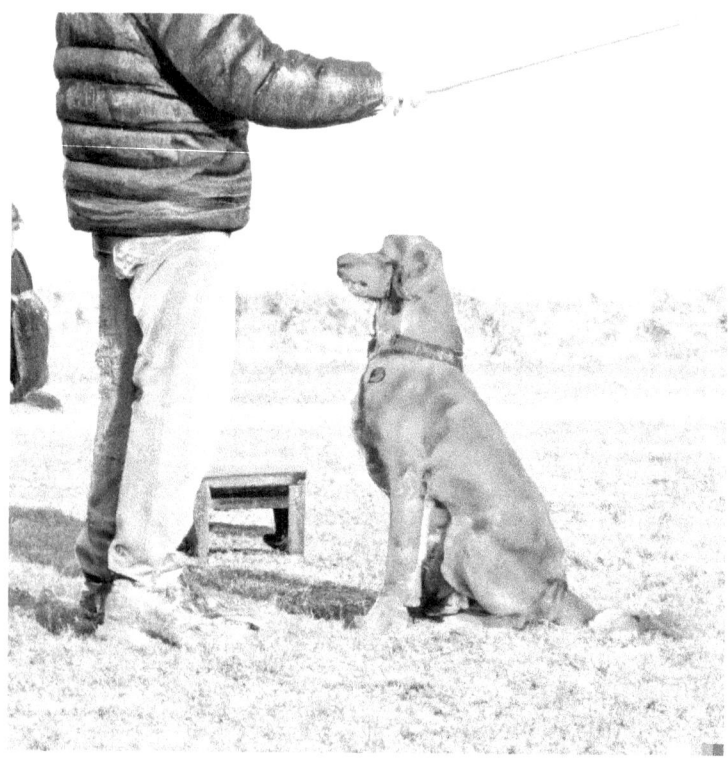

I am a dog lover, and I have always been fascinated by the intelligence and loyalty of dogs. I got my own dog, a Golden Retriever named Max, when he was just a few weeks old. At first, he was just a cute little bundle of fur, but as he grew older, I realized that he needed training to become a well-behaved and obedient dog.

Max was a lively and playful pup, but he had a mind of his own. He loved to jump on people, chew on things, and run around the house. At first, I thought it was just a phase and that he would grow out of it, but as he got bigger, his behavior became more problematic. He would jump on strangers, bark at the mailman, and destroy furniture. I realized that I needed to train him, but I didn't know where to start. I read books and watched videos, but I still felt overwhelmed. That's when I decided to hire a professional dog trainer. The trainer came to our house and spent several hours with us, teaching us how to train Max.

The first thing the trainer taught us was how to establish ourselves as the pack leader. We learned how to use positive reinforcement and gentle correction to teach Max what was acceptable behavior and what was not. We learned how to use treats and toys to motivate him, and how to use body language and tone of voice to communicate with him.

At first, Max resisted our training. He didn't like being told what to do, and he would often ignore our commands. But we persisted, and over time, he began to understand what we wanted from him. He learned how to sit, stay, and come when called. He learned how to walk on a leash without pulling, and how to greet people politely.

As Max became better trained, our relationship with him improved. He became more responsive to us, and we became more confident in our ability to handle him. We started taking him to public places, and he behaved well around people and other dogs.

The importance of training became clear when Max got loose from our yard one day. We searched frantically for him, but couldn't find him. Eventually, we got a call from a neighbor who had found Max several blocks away. He had been running around, and had almost caused a car accident.

When we got Max back, we realized how lucky we were that he hadn't been hurt. We also realized how important it was to have a well-trained dog. From that day forward, we made a commitment to continue Max's training, and to always be responsible dog owners.

In the end, the time and effort we spent training Max paid off in so many ways. We had a happy, well-behaved dog who was a joy to be around. We had a stronger bond with him, and we knew that he was safe and well-cared for. Training our dog was one of the best decisions we ever made, and we will always be grateful for the experience.

Training your dog is one of the most important things you can do as a pet owner. A well-trained dog is easier to manage, happier, and safer around people and other animals. Training your dog takes time and patience, but the rewards are well worth the effort. Here are some tips on how to train your dog effectively.

Start Early: The best time to start training your dog is when they are young. Puppies are like sponges and can learn quickly, so start teaching them basic commands such as sit, stay, and come as early as possible. This will help establish good habits early on and make training easier as your dog gets older.

Use Positive Reinforcement: Positive reinforcement is one of the most effective training techniques for dogs. This involves rewarding your dog for good behavior with treats, praise, or playtime. When your dog performs a desired behavior, immediately reward them to reinforce that behavior. Over time, your dog will learn that good behavior is rewarded and will be more likely to repeat it.

Be Consistent: Consistency is key when it comes to training your dog. Use the same commands and techniques each time you train, and make sure everyone in the household is on the same page. Inconsistency can confuse your dog and make training more difficult.

Keep Training Sessions Short: Dogs have short attention spans, so it's important to keep training sessions short and sweet. Ten to fifteen-minute sessions a few times a day are more effective than one long session. Keep the training sessions fun and engaging for your dog by incorporating playtime and treats.

Be Patient: Training your dog takes time and patience. Don't expect your dog to learn everything overnight. Be patient and take your time. If your dog is struggling with a particular behavior, break it down into smaller steps and reward each step of progress.

Consider Professional Help: If you're struggling with training your dog or if you have a particularly challenging dog, consider seeking help from a professional dog trainer. A trainer can help you identify problem areas and develop a customized training plan for your dog.

Final Thoughts: Training your dog is an essential part of being a responsible pet owner. Remember to start early, use positive reinforcement, be consistent, keep training sessions short, and be patient. With time and effort, you can train your dog to be a well-behaved and happy companion.

Dogs' Diseases and Symptoms

I woke up to the sound of my dog, Max, barking in distress. As I walked over to him, I could see that he was scratching himself relentlessly. His fur was coming out in clumps, and his skin was red and inflamed.

I didn't know what was wrong with him, so I decided to take him to the vet. As I explained Max's symptoms to the vet, I could sense a look of concern on their face. They asked me if I had recently changed his food or if he had been exposed to any new chemicals or substances. I couldn't think of anything that had changed, and I realized that I had not been paying close attention to his health in general.

The vet decided to run some tests, and it was then that I learned that Max had contracted a severe case of mange. I was shocked and horrified. I had never even heard of mange before. The vet explained that mange is a highly contagious skin disease caused by mites, and it is common in dogs that have weakened immune systems.

I was devastated. I couldn't believe that I had allowed this to happen to my beloved pet. The vet prescribed medication for Max, and we went home with a lot of instructions on how to care for him. I spent the next few weeks nursing Max back to health, making sure he got his medication on time, and taking extra precautions to prevent the spread of the disease to other dogs.

As Max recovered, I began to realize how much I had taken his health for granted. I had been ignorant of the signs that he was not feeling well, and I had not been proactive in keeping him healthy. I had let my guard down, and it had resulted in my poor dog contracting a severe illness.

I learned a valuable lesson that day. I realized that I needed to be more attentive to Max's health, to keep him up-to-date on his vaccinations, and to take him to the vet regularly. I vowed to do everything in my power to keep him healthy and happy, and I was grateful for the opportunity to make things right. Now, every time I see Max wag his tail and run around, I feel a sense of relief and gratitude. I know that he is healthy and happy again, and that I have learned a lesson that I will never forget.

Dogs are our beloved pets, and just like humans, they are prone to various health issues. There are several diseases that are common among dogs, and early detection and treatment can prevent them from becoming severe. In this article, we will discuss some of the most common dog diseases, their causes, and their symptoms.

- Canine Parvovirus: This is a highly contagious viral disease that affects puppies and unvaccinated dogs. It is spread through contact with infected feces, and symptoms include vomiting, diarrhea, loss of appetite, and lethargy.
- Canine Distemper: This is another viral disease that is highly contagious and can affect a dog's respiratory, gastrointestinal, and nervous systems. It

is spread through direct contact with infected body fluids, and symptoms include coughing, fever, diarrhea, and seizures.

- Kennel Cough: This is a respiratory infection that is caused by a combination of viruses and bacteria. It is highly contagious and can spread easily in environments where dogs are in close proximity to each other, such as kennels. Symptoms include coughing, sneezing, and a runny nose.
- Lyme Disease: This is a bacterial infection that is transmitted through tick bites. It affects dogs in various ways, including fever, joint pain, and loss of appetite. In severe cases, it can cause kidney damage.
- Canine Hepatitis: This is a viral disease that affects a dog's liver and can be spread through contact with infected urine, feces, or saliva. Symptoms include fever, vomiting, diarrhea, and loss of appetite.
- Canine Influenza: This is a respiratory infection that is caused by a virus and is highly contagious. It is spread through contact with infected dogs, and symptoms include coughing, fever, and lethargy.
- Heartworm Disease: This is a parasitic disease that is transmitted through mosquito bites. It affects a dog's heart and lungs and can be fatal if left untreated. Symptoms include coughing, difficulty breathing, and fatigue.

To prevent these diseases, it is important to keep your dog's vaccinations up to date, maintain good hygiene, and keep them away from infected animals. If you notice any of these symptoms in your dog, seek veterinary care immediately to prevent the disease from becoming severe.

Dogs are prone to various diseases, and early detection and treatment are crucial in preventing them from becoming severe. It is important to keep your dog's vaccinations up to date, maintain good hygiene, and keep them away from infected animals to prevent the spread of these diseases.

Taking Care of Your Dog

Dogs are often considered to be a man's best friend. They are loyal, loving, and always there to provide companionship. As a pet owner, it is important to ensure that your furry friend is happy and healthy. Here are some tips on taking care of your dog pet:

Proper Nutrition: Just like humans, dogs require a balanced and nutritious diet to stay healthy. Ensure that your dog's diet consists of high-quality dog food that is rich in protein and nutrients. Avoid feeding your dog table scraps, as it may cause digestive issues and lead to obesity.

Regular Exercise: Exercise is crucial for a dog's physical and mental well-being. Ensure that your dog gets enough exercise every day. Take them for walks, play with them in the backyard, or take them to the dog park.

Regular Vet Checkups: Regular visits to the veterinarian are essential for maintaining your dog's health. Ensure that your dog is up-to-date on all their vaccinations, and visit the vet immediately if you notice any signs of illness or discomfort.

Proper Grooming: Grooming your dog is not just about keeping them looking good. It also helps maintain their health. Regularly brush your dog's coat to prevent matting and shedding. Bathe your dog when necessary, and trim their nails to prevent them from growing too long.

Provide a Safe Environment: Dogs love to explore and play, but it is important to provide them with a safe environment. Keep toxic substances out of reach, secure gates and doors to prevent them from running away, and provide a comfortable and safe sleeping area.

Training and Socialization: Training and socialization are essential for a dog's behavior and mental health. Ensure that your dog is trained to obey basic commands, and socialize them with other dogs and people.

Show Them Love and Affection: Dogs thrive on love and attention. Spend time with your dog, play with them, and show them affection in a way that they enjoy. This can include petting them, giving them belly rubs, or playing with their favorite toy. When you show your dog love and affection, they will feel happy and secure, which can improve their overall well-being and strengthen the bond between you and your furry friend.

Dogs also benefit from regular exercise and mental stimulation, so make sure to take your dog for walks, play fetch with them, or engage them in interactive games. These activities not only provide physical exercise, but also help to stimulate your dog's mind and prevent boredom.

In addition to spending time with your dog, it's important to provide them with a safe and comfortable living environment. This includes providing them with a cozy bed, clean water, and healthy food. You should also ensure that your dog receives regular veterinary check-ups and preventative care to keep them healthy and happy.

Overall, showing love and affection to your dog is an important part of being a responsible and caring pet owner. By spending time with your furry friend, playing with them, and providing them with a safe and comfortable living environment, you can help ensure that they live a happy and healthy life.

www.ingramcontent.com/pod-product-compliance
Lightning Source LLC
Chambersburg PA
CBHW070750220526
45467CB00018B/1855